AORTIC VALVE STENOSIS

I0422221

Diagnosis, Treatment, and Living a Heart-Healthy Life with Aortic Valve Stenosis: A Comprehensive Guide

CARL JUAN

Table of Contents

Introductory

The aortic valve in the heart can become narrowed due to a medical disease known as aortic stenosis. The aortic valve is one of the heart's four valves, controlling the flow of blood from the heart into the aorta. The aorta is the body's largest artery, transporting oxygen-rich blood to the rest of the body. By definition, aortic stenosis is a narrowing or constriction of the aortic valve that prevents blood from flowing freely from the heart's left ventricle into the aorta.

• In most cases, calcium deposits on the valve leaflets over time cause the aortic valve to narrow and become less able to open and close normally. Symptoms such as chest pain, shortness of breath, exhaustion, and fainting might develop because the heart has to work harder to pump blood through the constricted valve. Aortic valve stenosis can lead to life-threatening problems like cardiac failure in extreme circumstances.

Medication can be used to treat symptoms and track the progression of aortic valve stenosis. To restore normal blood flow and relieve the obstruction, surgical treatments such as aortic valve replacement or repair may be required in more severe situations. Aortic valve stenosis is a degenerative illness, and early identification and care are critical for achieving the best possible outcomes for patients.

CHAPTER ONE
How the Aortic Valve Is Built and How It Works

One of the four heart valves responsible for controlling blood flow is the aortic valve. It is situated between the body's biggest artery (the aorta) and the left ventricle (the heart's main pumping chamber). The aortic valve's form and function are crucial to the health of the heart as a whole.

The Aortic Valve's Internal Structure

• The aortic valve has three leaflets, or cusps, that are thin, pliable, and triangular in shape. The aortic valve's leaflets are rings of tough, fibrous tissue that are connected to the valve's annulus. The aortic valve's leaflets open and close to regulate blood flow from the left ventricle into the aorta.

To What End Does the Aortic Valve Exist?

• The aortic valve's main job is to regulate blood flow, making sure that oxygenated blood is pushed from the left ventricle into the aorta and subsequently out to the rest of the body. This valve allows blood to flow from the left ventricle into the aorta during systole, when the heart is contracting.

- **Preventing Backflow**: The aortic valve's leaflets are designed to seal tightly during the heart's relaxation phase (diastole) to prevent blood from flowing back into the left ventricle. Blood with high oxygen levels and blood with low oxygen levels are kept apart by the heart's one-way valves.

- By controlling blood flow into the aorta, the aortic valve keeps the body's oxygenated blood circulating to all of its organs and tissues, where it can provide vital nutrients and oxygen for healthy functioning.

The electrical and mechanical activity of the heart are exactly timed with the opening and closing of the aortic valve. Aortic valve stenosis (narrowing) and aortic valve regurgitation (leakage) are two of the many aortic valve disorders that can cause a variety of heart problems and necessitate medical intervention to restore normal valve function.

The unidirectional flow of blood from the heart to the body, which is maintained by the aortic valve, is essential for the normal functioning of all of the body's organs and tissues, including the brain.

Regular Operation of Valves

The four heart valves open and close in unison to allow blood to travel in just one direction through the heart and the rest of the body's circulatory system. The four heart valves are the aortic valve, mitral valve, tricuspid valve, and pulmonary valve. The typical operation of a valve is as follows:

• The aortic valve, also known as the semilunar valve, connects the left ventricle to the aorta, the body's main artery. The aortic valve opens as the left ventricle contracts (systole) during the cardiac cycle. To deliver oxygenated blood to the remainder of the body, the left ventricle pumps blood into the aorta. The aortic valve seals off the left ventricle from the aorta when the left ventricle relaxes (diastole).

• The bicuspid mitral valve separates the left atrium (upper chamber) from the left ventricle (lower chamber). The mitral valve opens during diastole to allow blood to flow from the left atrium into the left ventricle. The mitral valve seals off the left atrium from the left ventricle when the left ventricle contracts during systole.

• The tricuspid valve is the one connecting the right atrium to the right ventricle. Like the mitral valve, it opens when the right atrium contracts during diastole and shuts when the right ventricle contracts during systole.

• The pulmonary valve, also known as the semilunar valve, is located between the right ventricle and the pulmonary artery, the blood vessel responsible for transporting oxygen-depleted blood from the heart to the lungs. The pulmonary valve opens and blood is pushed into the pulmonary artery during systole, when the right ventricle contracts. During diastole, when the right ventricle is at rest, the pulmonary valve closes to seal off the ventricle from the pulmonary artery.

Maintaining unidirectional blood flow through the heart, preventing the mixing of oxygenated and deoxygenated blood, and guaranteeing effective distribution of blood to the body's organs and tissues all depend on the regular functioning of these heart valves. Medical intervention or surgical repair may be necessary to restore normal valve function in cases of stenosis (narrowing), regurgitation (leakage), or prolapse, all of which can cause heart-related complications. The heart's ability to pump blood efficiently and sustain cardiovascular health relies on the proper functioning of its valves.

CHAPTER TWO
Valve Health and Its Determinants

Valve health in the heart can be influenced by different variables, and maintaining the normal functioning of heart valves is critical for overall cardiovascular health. The condition of a valve can be affected by the following:

• Heart valve performance can be impaired by age-related degeneration and loss of pliability. Aortic valve stenosis and mitral valve regurgitation are two disorders that can develop as people age.

- Heart valve abnormalities and congenital heart problems can have a significant impact on a person's quality of life. Surgical intervention may be necessary to fix these issues.

- **Infections:** Valve infections, such as infective endocarditis, can damage heart valves. Inflammation and damage to heart valves can result from bacterial or fungal infections.

- **Rheumatic Fever:** This condition, brought on by untreated streptococcal throat infections, can scar and damage heart valves, most notably the mitral and aortic valves.

• Aortic valve stenosis is a condition in which the aortic valve narrows and blood flow is restricted because of a buildup of calcium deposits on the valve leaflets.

• **High Blood Pressure (Hypertension)**: High blood pressure can lead to greater stress on the heart valves, potentially leading them to thicken and weaken over time.

• Abnormalities in the structure of the heart valves can lead to a variety of conditions known together as valvular heart disease. These issues can also develop over time or be present at birth.

• Aortic valve stenosis is caused by atherosclerosis, which is characterized by the buildup of fatty deposits and plaques on the aortic valve.

• Inflammation and damage to heart valves have been linked to autoimmune illnesses including systemic lupus erythematosus.

• Some medications, including those used to treat Parkinson's disease and some weight reduction aids, have been linked to an increased risk of valvular heart disease.

• Radiation therapy is commonly used to treat cancer, but it can cause serious complications to the heart, including damage to the heart valves.

• Mitral valve health is particularly vulnerable to hormonal changes brought on by pregnancy, menopause, or hormone replacement therapy.

• **Smoking:** Smoking and exposure to tobacco smoke are risk factors for cardiovascular disease, including valve difficulties.

• **Obesity:** Being overweight or obese increases your risk of developing a number of cardiovascular conditions, including issues with your heart valves.

For optimal cardiovascular health, it's crucial to take care of your heart's valves. The risk of valve problems can be lowered by adopting a healthy lifestyle, which includes eating right, exercising frequently, not smoking, and controlling illnesses like high blood pressure and diabetes. Valve health can be maintained with routine doctor visits and the correct medical management of heart issues. Heart valves that have been compromised may require surgical intervention.

Changes in the structure and function of the aortic valve and the heart are at the root of the pathophysiology of aortic valve stenosis. When the aortic valve becomes stenotic, blood cannot efficiently move from the left ventricle of the heart into the body's main blood vessel, the aorta. Because of this blockage, left ventricular pressure rises, which can have a number of adverse effects:

• Aortic valve stenosis begins with a thickening and calcification of the aortic valve leaflets, a valvular alteration. Calcium deposits harden and reduce the pliability of the valve leaflets over time. Because of this, the valve can't open all the way during systole (when the ventricles contract) and close all the way during diastole (when the ventricles relax).

• Reduced blood flow because the aortic valve's aperture (opening) becomes smaller as its leaflets become stiffer. As a result of this constriction, the heart has to work harder to pump blood from the left ventricle into the aorta during systole.

• The left ventricle enlarges because it must pump blood at a higher pressure during systole to overcome the increased resistance generated by the constricted aortic valve. The left ventricular wall thickens (hypertrophy) in response to this increased pressure. Left ventricular hypertrophy is the heart's attempt to maintain normal cardiac output by contracting more strongly.

• Left ventricular hypertrophy raises the threshold at which the heart's muscle requires oxygen. This can raise your likelihood of experiencing angina (chest discomfort) or other symptoms related to ischemia (inadequate blood flow) in the heart muscle.

• Decreased cardiac output occurs because of the left ventricle's decreasing efficiency when aortic valve stenosis worsens. Reduced cardiac output can cause weariness, shortness of breath, and an inability to tolerate physical exertion, among other symptoms.

• Heart pressure overload: long-term increased stress on the heart's left ventricle can cause heart failure. If the left ventricle enlarges and loses its pumping efficiency, cardiac output will drop even further.

• To keep blood flowing, the body may use compensating strategies, such as a faster heart rate and stronger cardiac contractions. These processes may place additional strain on the heart while they attempt to compensate for the stenosis.

• In terms of clinical symptoms, stenosis can cause chest pain, shortness of breath, dizziness, and weariness as it progresses. Syncope (temporary loss of consciousness) and abrupt cardiac death are two of the potentially fatal side effects of severe aortic valve stenosis.

Aortic valve stenosis is a serious condition that need immediate attention due to the pathophysiology involved. Once the issue becomes severe and symptomatic, surgical procedures, such as aortic valve replacement, are typically necessary to remove the obstruction and restore normal blood flow through the aortic valve, thereby improving the patient's overall cardiovascular health. Aortic valve stenosis can lead to serious health problems in the road, so it's important to catch it early and treat it so it doesn't become worse.

CHAPTER THREE
The Development of the Illness

The worsening of aortic valve stenosis typically takes place over the course of several years. The rate at which aortic valve stenosis, the narrowing of the aortic valve, progresses varies from patient to patient.

• In the early stages of aortic valve stenosis, the patient may not have any symptoms. This is known as the asymptomatic phase. However, aberrant valve structure or function can be picked up by diagnostic techniques like echocardiography, which can identify the presence of aortic valve stenosis.

• Aortic valve stenosis may be modest at first, causing just a slight restriction of blood flow. The heart may frequently compensate for the slight restriction by raising the force of contraction to maintain normal blood flow.

• Over time, the stenosis may worsen to a moderate degree, which is the most common clinical presentation. Left ventricular hypertrophy (thickening of the left ventricular wall) continues to occur as the heart adjusts to sustain cardiac output. Patients may have no symptoms at this point.

• Patients may experience symptoms when the stenosis worsens and the aortic valve's orifice becomes considerably narrowed, a phase known as the symptomatic phase. Angina chest pain, weariness, inability to exercise, and shortness of breath are all common symptoms. These signs and symptoms originate from the decreased cardiac output and increased workload on the left ventricle.

• Aortic stenosis becomes so severe that the heart can no longer adequately compensate for the restriction. The left ventricle may weaken and cardiac output may decrease. Left untreated, this stage of the disease can lead to heart failure, which may present as symptoms including fluid retention (edema) and shortness of breath at rest.

• Syncope (passing out), arrhythmias, and sudden cardiac death are only few of the consequences that can arise from severe aortic valve stenosis. Significant hemodynamic abnormalities may be linked with these problems, making prompt medical care essential.

It is not always possible to predict how quickly or slowly aortic valve stenosis will worsen in any given individual. Age, the etiology of the stenosis, and the existence of other heart diseases are just a few of the factors that can affect how quickly the disease progresses. The best way to improve the patient's quality of life and prevent complications is to catch the problem early through regular checkups and appropriate monitoring of aortic valve function, so that aortic valve replacement, for example, can be performed before the condition worsens.

Aortic Valve Stenosis: Symptoms and Signs

Aortic stenosis is a narrowing of the aortic valve that prevents blood from flowing freely from the heart's left ventricle into the aorta. The symptoms of stenosis may not present themselves until the disease has progressed to a more severe stage. Aortic valve stenosis symptoms typically include:

• Patients with aortic valve stenosis may not suffer any symptoms in the early stages, known as the asymptomatic phase. Regular checkups and diagnostic procedures could reveal the illness.

• **Chest Pain (Angina):** As the stenosis progresses, some persons may experience chest pain or discomfort, especially during physical exercise or exertion. When the aortic valve is blocked, the heart has to work harder to get the oxygen it needs, resulting in angina.

• One of the most prevalent signs of aortic valve stenosis is dyspnea, or shortness of breath. While it is most common during exercise, the illness can also manifest itself while at rest or while sleeping. The diminished ability of the heart to pump blood can lead to an accumulation of fluid in the lungs, producing dyspnea.

• Aortic valve stenosis patients may feel fatigued and unable to carry out their regular routines. As a result of the increased effort required by the heart to pump blood through the constricted valve, patients may experience fatigue.

• Loss of Consciousness (Syncope): Some people with severe aortic valve stenosis may have syncopal episodes. Inadequate blood supply to the brain from the heart can cause this.

• An abnormal cardiac murmur might be heard by a doctor during a physical examination. A constricted aortic valve causes turbulent blood flow, which can be heard as a murmur.

• In some people with aortic valve stenosis, irregular heartbeats or palpitations may develop. Arrhythmias, caused by stress on the heart, have been linked to these abnormal heartbeats.

It's crucial to remember that not everyone with aortic valve stenosis will suffer the same symptoms or have the same disease progression. Aortic valve stenosis can cause heart failure, arrhythmias, and even abrupt cardiac death in extreme situations. Patients with aortic valve stenosis benefit greatly from prompt diagnosis and treatment, which may include aortic valve replacement surgery. If you or someone you know is suffering any of these symptoms, it's crucial to seek medical examination and counsel from a healthcare expert.

Evaluation and Diagnostic Procedures

Aortic valve stenosis is evaluated and diagnosed after a thorough medical history is taken, a physical examination is performed, and a battery of diagnostic testing is performed. These aid doctors in determining the stenosis's degree, evaluating its effects on the heart, and deciding on a course of treatment. Aortic valve stenosis is evaluated and diagnosed with the following methods:

1. Physical Examining and Medical History:

• The patient should expect to be asked about symptoms, risk factors, and previous heart issues as part of the healthcare provider's in-depth medical history.

• A physical examination will be undertaken to listen for typical heart murmurs linked with aortic stenosis and check general health.

2. Echocardiography:

• Aortic valve stenosis is most commonly diagnosed with transthoracic echocardiography (TTE), a type of echocardiography.

To evaluate the heart and its aortic valve, transthoracic echocardiography (TTE) employs the use of high-frequency sound waves (ultrasound).

• It shows how much the valve has shrunk, how thick the leaflets are, and if there is any regurgitation (leakage).

3. A Doppler Echocardiogram:

• Doppler echocardiography is typically used in conjunction with TTE to assess blood flow velocity and pressure gradients across the aortic valve.

• The severity of aortic stenosis and its effect on blood flow can be gauged with the use of this diagnostic tool.

4. Echocardiography Performed Through the Throat (TEE):

• To improve the quality of cardiac imaging, including the aortic valve, TEE uses a specialized probe placed into the esophagus.

• When TTE findings are ambiguous, or when more detailed pictures are required, this technique may be employed.

5. ECG or EKG (electrocardiogram):

• Rhythm irregularities or evidence of left ventricular hypertrophy can be detected with the aid of an electrocardiogram (ECG).

6. An X-ray of the chest:

• Heart size and shape, as well as fluid in the lungs and symptoms of heart failure, can all be seen on a chest X-ray.

7. Catheterization of the Heart:

• Cardiac catheterization may be conducted to directly monitor pressure in the heart chambers and examine the severity of aortic stenosis.

• If valve replacement is in the works, it can also be used to evaluate the severity of coronary artery disease and whether or not bypass surgery is required.

8. The Stress of Exercise:

Aortic stenosis patients can learn more about how exercise affects their symptoms and heart function with a stress test.

9. (Magnetic Resonance Imaging) Cardiac MRI:

• Cardiac MRI can evaluate valve function and other aspects of heart health by providing comprehensive images of the heart.

• It can be utilized when more data is required or when other diagnostic methods come up empty.

10. Analyzing Biomarkers:

• Biomarkers such brain natriuretic peptide (BNP) and N-terminal pro b-type natriuretic peptide (NT-proBNP) can be measured in the blood to aid in the diagnosis and evaluation of heart failure.

The clinical presentation of the patient and the discretion of the healthcare professional are primary considerations in selecting appropriate diagnostic tests. The findings of these tests help evaluate the severity of aortic valve stenosis and guide treatment options, such as the time and type of intervention, which may involve aortic valve replacement surgery. The severity of the illness and its effects on the heart can only be gauged with consistent monitoring and follow-up.

CHAPTER FOUR
Evaluation and Categorization

The pressure gradient across the aortic valve and the aortic valve area are used to categorize and evaluate the severity of aortic valve stenosis. Echocardiography and Doppler measures are the gold standards for assessing and categorizing aortic valve stenosis. American College of Cardiology/American Heart Association (ACC/AHA) and European Society of Cardiology (ESC) classifications are the two most widely used systems for evaluating aortic stenosis severity.

1. Classification by the American Heart Association and the American College of Cardiology (ACC/AHA):

• Aortic stenosis is classified into three phases by the ACC/AHA: mild, moderate, and severe.

• There is no detectable aortic valve stenosis in Stage A. Patients without aortic stenosis may have risk factors for the disorder, such as a bicuspid aortic valve.

• Asymptomatic patients with echocardiographic evidence of mild to moderate aortic stenosis are classified as being in Stage B.

- **Phase C:** This phase is broken down into three distinct phases:

Patients at this stage have significant aortic stenosis but no symptoms.

- Chest pain (angina), shortness of breath, and exercise intolerance are all signs of stage C2 aortic stenosis.

Aortic stenosis is regarded to be low-flow, low-gradient when it reaches the stage C3 and the patient is suffering symptoms.

2. It is classified as such by the ESC (European Society of Cardiology).

Aortic stenosis is evaluated according to the ESC classification system by evaluating many echocardiographic parameters.

- Aortic valve stenosis is not present in Stage 0.

When the aortic valve area is more than or equal to 1.5 cm2, mild aortic stenosis is present.

- **Stage 2**: aortic stenosis is characterized by an aortic valve area of 1.0 cm2 to 1.5 cm2.

- **Stage 3:** Severe aortic stenosis with an aortic valve area less than 1.0 cm^2.

Stage 4: Extremely narrow aortic opening, as measured by a very low stroke volume index and a mean pressure gradient of less than 40 mm Hg.

Aortic valve stenosis severity is assessed and treatment decisions are made using both the ACC/AHA and ESC criteria. Factors such as left ventricular function and the patient's overall health, as well as the severity of the stenosis and the presence of symptoms, play a role in determining whether or not aortic valve replacement surgery is warranted. The only way to track the development of a disease and intervene effectively when needed is through consistent monitoring and follow-up.

Relieving Symptoms with Medication

Although aortic valve replacement is the gold standard treatment for severe aortic valve stenosis, medications can be used to help manage symptoms and improve the patient's quality of life, particularly if the patient is not an immediate surgical candidate or if the surgical procedure must be delayed.

1. Medication to Reduce Angina:

• Nitroglycerin helps reduce the strain on the heart and alleviates chest pain (angina) by widening blood vessels. Patients with aortic stenosis who are experiencing angina may get symptomatic alleviation from this treatment.

2. Diuretics:

• Fluid retention and heart failure symptoms like dyspnea and swelling can be managed with the help of diuretics such loop diuretics (like furosemide).

3. Beta-Blockers:

- Beta-blockers (e.g., metoprolol, carvedilol) can reduce the oxygen demand of the heart muscle and lower the heart rate. They are sometimes used for symptom control and to ease chest discomfort.

4. Antihypertensive Drugs:

- Medication to reduce blood pressure, such as angiotensin-converting enzyme (ACE) inhibitors or angiotensin receptor blockers (ARBs), may be recommended.

5. Medication for Arrhythmia:

• To control the potentially life-threatening arrhythmias that might arise in patients with severe aortic stenosis, antiarrhythmic medicines such as amiodarone may be prescribed.

6. Statins:

• Cholesterol-lowering drugs called statins (including atorvastatin and simvastatin) may be recommended to patients with aortic stenosis to help alleviate the symptoms of atherosclerosis and coronary artery disease, which are often present in patients with aortic stenosis.

7. In severe situations, inotropes:

- Intravenous inotropes (such as dobutamine): intravenous inotropes may be used to temporarily improve heart function and hemodynamics in critically ill individuals with severe heart failure.

Even though these drugs can alleviate symptoms and boost a patient's quality of life, they don't address what's causing aortic valve stenosis in the first place. Ultimately, the definitive treatment for severe aortic stenosis is aortic valve replacement, which can be performed surgically or via less invasive procedures such as transcatheter aortic valve replacement (TAVR). The severity of the stenosis, the presence of symptoms, and the patient's general health all play a role in determining when the valve replacement should take place. Patients with severe aortic stenosis should check in with their doctors on a regular basis to discuss their symptoms and treatment options.

CHAPTER FIVE

Changing One's Way of Life and Preventing Disease

While medical and surgical treatments are the mainstays of aortic valve stenosis management, disease modification and lifestyle changes can aid in overall heart health and may even halt the progression of the problem. In the early stages of aortic valve stenosis or as part of a holistic strategy for heart health, these interventions can be helpful for patients. Some suggestions are as follows:

1. Checking in with a doctor on a regular basis is crucial for keeping tabs on how your aortic valve stenosis is progressing. Regular checkups make it possible to identify any subtle changes in the health and respond swiftly.

2. Blood Pressure Management: Keeping blood pressure within a healthy range is crucial. Aortic stenosis may worsen due to the added strain that high blood pressure places on the heart. Adjustments to one's way of life, together with medication if necessary, can help keep blood pressure in check.

3. Cholesterol Management: Lowering the risk of atherosclerosis (the hardening and narrowing of the arteries) requires attention to one's cholesterol levels, in particular one's LDL ("bad") cholesterol. Cholesterol levels can be managed with dietary changes and statin medicines.

4. Moderate exercise on a regular basis is associated with improved heart health. Individuals with severe aortic stenosis should consult a healthcare provider for advice on the appropriate level of exercise, as excessive physical stress can exacerbate the condition.

5. Fruits, vegetables, whole grains, lean proteins, and a diet low in saturated and trans fats are all part of a heart-healthy diet. Sodium restriction can also aid in the control of hypertension and fluid retention.

6. Quitting smoking is one of the most important things smokers can do for their heart health. Aortic stenosis, like many other forms of cardiovascular disease, is greatly exacerbated by smoking.

7. Controlling One's Weight: • Being at a healthy weight has been shown to lessen stress on the heart and improve cardiovascular health.

8. Reducing stress: long-term stress has been linked to heart disease. Engaging in stress reduction techniques such as meditation, deep breathing, or yoga can be beneficial.

9. Adherence to prescribed medication is essential if you have been diagnosed with a condition that necessitates treatment with medication, such as high blood pressure, high cholesterol, or diabetes.

10. Prevention of Valve-Related Endocarditis through Proper Dental Hygiene Infections, including those that occur in the mouth, can increase the risk of valve-related endocarditis.

11. Schedule regular dental checkups and practice good oral hygiene to reduce your risk of developing endocarditis.

12. Vaccines: People with heart valve conditions should be sure to get all of their recommended vaccinations, including the flu shot and pneumococcal vaccine.

Although these interventions may improve cardiac health and aid in the management of secondary conditions, they will not cure aortic valve stenosis. Aortic valve replacement is the gold standard treatment for severe aortic stenosis, which is usually recommended when symptoms appear. The severity of stenosis, the presence of symptoms, and the patient's general health all play a role in deciding when valve replacement should take place. Always seek the counsel of a medical professional for specific recommendations tailored to your needs.

Continued Treatment and Evaluation

Aortic valve stenosis patients must be followed and monitored to determine how far along the disease process they are, how severe their symptoms are, and how best to proceed with treatment. Aortic stenosis patients may require different amounts and types of follow-up care, depending on the severity of their condition and their own unique circumstances. Care and monitoring after aortic valve stenosis surgery should focus on the following areas:

• Patients with aortic stenosis should see a cardiologist or cardiac surgeon on a regular basis. The recommended minimum interval between visits is one year; however, this may vary depending on the severity of the stenosis, the presence of symptoms, and other factors.

• Ultrasound of the heart (echocardiography) is a crucial diagnostic tool for monitoring the health of the aortic valve. This examination is useful for diagnosing stenosis and tracking its progression over time.

• A patient's symptoms, such as chest pain, shortness of breath, fatigue, or fainting, will be evaluated during a visit to the doctor. When to replace an aortic valve depends heavily on the severity and duration of symptoms.

• An electrocardiogram (ECG or EKG) may be performed during checkups to detect arrhythmias or other electrical abnormalities in the heart and track their progression over time.

• Aortic stenosis can worsen with hypertension, so it's crucial to measure blood pressure regularly. It's crucial to keep blood pressure readings within a healthy range.

• Care providers will assess patients' dietary and exercise habits, as well as their adherence to prescribed medications, to guarantee that their patients are implementing the best practices for preventing and treating cardiovascular disease.

• Patients with valvular heart disease should be informed of their diagnosis, potential treatments, and side effects. When patients have a firm grasp on their condition, they are better able to take an active role in their treatment.

• Consultation with cardiac surgeons to determine the best time for aortic valve replacement, either through traditional open-heart surgery or minimally invasive techniques like transcatheter aortic valve replacement (TAVR), may be part of the aftercare plan for patients with severe aortic stenosis.

• Adjustments to a patient's medication regimen may be made in response to evolving clinical and therapeutic circumstances. Symptoms can be controlled by modifying the dosages of various medications, such as diuretics, beta-blockers, and anti-anginal drugs.

• Cardiac magnetic resonance imaging (MRI) and computed tomography (CT) scans are examples of advanced imaging modalities that may be used to learn more about the heart's anatomy and physiology.

- After aortic valve replacement, either surgically or transcatheterally, it is crucial to conduct a risk assessment. Symptoms, left ventricular function, and the patient's overall health all play a role in determining whether or not intervention is necessary due to stenosis.

- Antibiotic prophylaxis for infective endocarditis is sometimes recommended for patients with aortic stenosis prior to undergoing specific dental or medical procedures.

Appropriate management of aortic valve stenosis requires consistent and regular follow-up care so that the optimal time for interventions like aortic valve replacement can be determined. Appointments should be kept, changes in lifestyle should be implemented, and medications and treatments should be taken exactly as prescribed by doctors.

CHAPTER SIX
Methods of Intervention and Surgical Treatment

When aortic valve stenosis is severe and causing symptoms, the only options for treatment are interventional and surgical. The patient's overall health, the presence of comorbid conditions, and the unique characteristics of the aortic valve stenosis all play a role in determining the best course of treatment. Aortic valve stenosis can be treated with the following interventional and surgical methods:

1. Replacement of the Aortic Valve (AVR):

• Aortic valve replacement is the most common and effective treatment for severe aortic valve stenosis.

• To restore healthy blood flow, AVR involves surgically removing the diseased aortic valve and replacing it with a mechanical valve (made of long-lasting materials) or a biological valve (typically from a pig or cow).

Open-chest surgery and less invasive procedures like transcatheter aortic valve replacement (TAVR) are both viable options for aortic valve replacement (AVR).

2. Aortic valve replacement using a catheter (TAVR):

• TAVR is a less invasive procedure used to replace the aortic valve in select patients, particularly those who are at higher risk for complications from open-heart surgery.

• Transcatheter aortic valve replacement (TAVR) eliminates the need for open-heart surgery by guiding a catheter through a blood vessel directly to the heart, where a new valve is implanted within the damaged aortic valve.

Patients with severe aortic stenosis who are deemed too high-risk for open-heart surgery may be candidates for TAVR.

3. Valvuloplasty Using a Balloon:

• Since it is not a permanent solution, balloon valvuloplasty is reserved for patients who are not surgical candidates.

• A balloon-tipped catheter is inflated inside the narrowed aortic valve to expand the valve opening in this procedure. However, the benefits typically only last temporarily, and the valve will eventually become less open again.

4. Waiting Cautiously:

• Mild or moderate aortic stenosis may not always call for emergency surgery. They are observed carefully, and treatment is given serious thought only if the stenosis worsens or if symptoms appear.

The presence and severity of symptoms, the patient's general health and age, and other medical factors all play a role in determining whether or not intervention or surgery is recommended. In order to choose the best course of treatment, patients must have in-depth conversations with their doctors and heart specialists.

After valve replacement, patients typically experience significant improvement in symptoms and overall quality of life. However, post-operative care and follow-up are essential for checking in on the patient's progress, gauging the effectiveness of the new valve, and making sure the patient is healthy overall. To aid in a speedy recovery and ensure long-term heart health, patients must take medications as prescribed and participate in a cardiac rehabilitation program.

Problems and Expectations

If aortic valve stenosis isn't treated, it can cause a host of serious complications. One's outlook after being diagnosed with aortic valve stenosis depends on the severity of the condition, the presence of symptoms, and the promptness with which treatment is administered. A few potential complications and their outlooks are listed below.

• Aortic valve stenosis can be so severe that it causes heart failure. Fluid retention, shortness of breath, and fatigue are all symptoms that may develop as the heart's ability to pump blood becomes compromised. Heart failure caused by aortic stenosis can have a grim prognosis if not treated properly.

• Syncope (fainting) and stroke are just two of the complications that can arise from arrhythmias, which are caused by aortic stenosis. Additional treatment and monitoring may be necessary for arrhythmias.

• Infective endocarditis, or an infection of the heart valves, is more common in people with heart valve abnormalities such as aortic stenosis. If not promptly treated, endocarditis can lead to severe complications and may have a poor prognosis.

• Aortic stenosis can cause decreased blood flow to the brain, which can cause syncope (temporary loss of consciousness) in some patients. Individuals experiencing syncope have varying prognoses depending on the etiology and treatment time of their condition.

• Increased risk of sudden cardiac death has been linked to severe aortic stenosis. Severe, symptomatic stenosis and underlying heart conditions are typically associated with this danger. Patients experiencing sudden cardiac death have a very poor prognosis and need emergency medical attention right away.

• Embolic strokes can occur as a result of aortic stenosis because of the increased likelihood of blood clot formation in the heart. Depending on the severity and location of the stroke, the prognosis for individuals who have suffered a stroke can vary significantly.

• Aortic stenosis tends to worsen over time if treatment isn't provided. The prognosis worsens with increasing stenosis severity, particularly in patients who exhibit severe symptoms.

In severe cases, aortic valve replacement is the only treatment option, but it greatly improves the prognosis for patients with aortic valve stenosis. Once the stenosed valve is replaced, patients typically experience relief from symptoms, improved quality of life, and a reduced risk of complications. In many cases, a better prognosis can be expected if treatment begins as soon as possible after symptoms appear.

Close monitoring is essential for people with mild or moderate aortic stenosis who are asymptomatic, as disease progression may eventually require intervention. Appropriate treatment timing can be determined and heart health can be maintained with regular follow-up with healthcare providers and cardiac specialists.

When aortic valve stenosis is diagnosed at an early stage and the necessary treatments are administered, the prognosis for the disease and its complications improves.

Conclusion

Aortic stenosis is a narrowing of the aortic valve that prevents blood from flowing freely from the left ventricle into the aorta, causing a variety of serious health problems. If untreated, it can worsen over time and cause symptoms like chest pain, shortness of breath, fatigue, and even heart failure. Evaluation of the patient's medical history, a physical examination, and a battery of diagnostic tests—including echocardiography all contribute to the diagnosis of aortic valve stenosis.

- Transcatheter aortic valve replacement (TAVR) and open-heart surgery are two options for treating aortic stenosis, but the former is the more common of the two. Medications are an option for symptom management, and healthy lifestyle choices can have a positive impact on cardiovascular health.

If patients with aortic valve stenosis are to have the best possible outcomes, they must receive consistent follow-up care, monitoring, and timely intervention. The choice of treatment and the timing of intervention depend on factors such as the severity of the stenosis, the presence of symptoms, and the patient's overall health. Early detection, appropriate medical care, and adherence to medical advice can help improve the quality of life and prognosis for individuals with aortic valve stenosis.

THE END